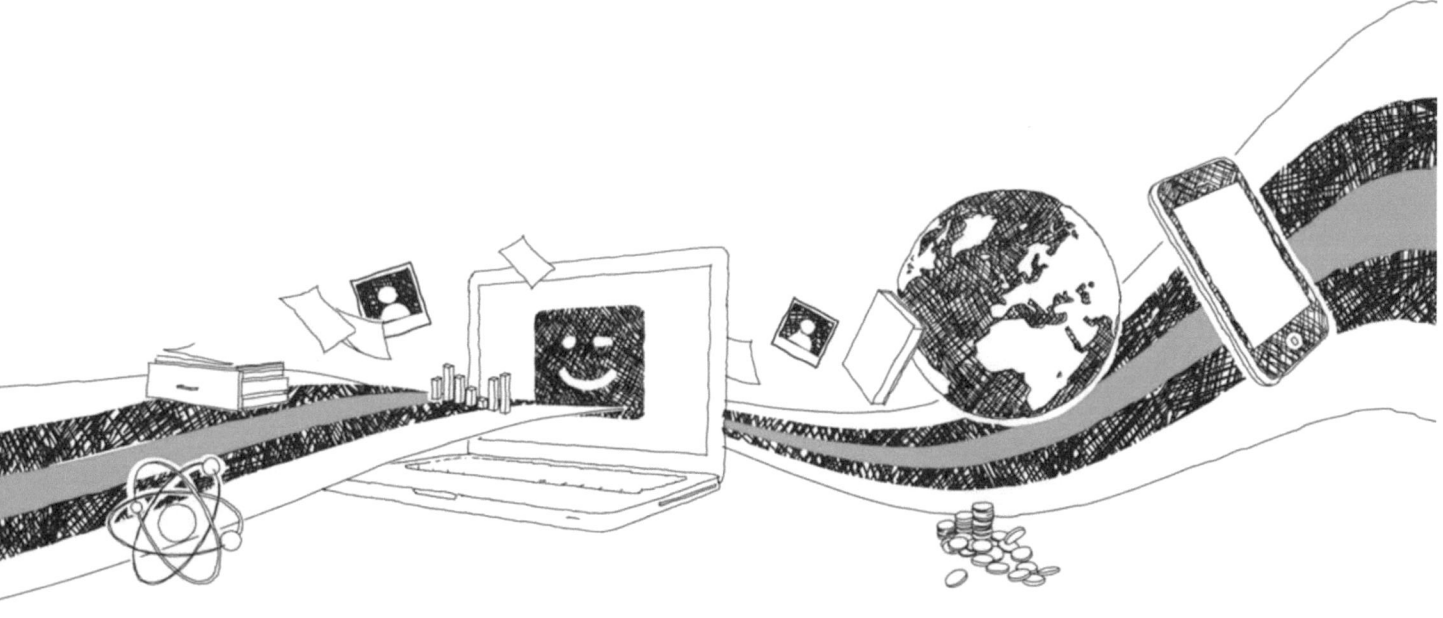
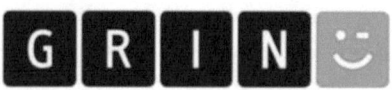

Clinton Kelly

Medical Marijuana and the Need for Regulation

GRIN Publishing

Bibliographic information published by the German National Library:

The German National Library lists this publication in the National Bibliography; detailed bibliographic data are available on the Internet at http://dnb.dnb.de .

Imprint:

Copyright © 2012 GRIN Verlag, Open Publishing GmbH
Print and binding: Books on Demand GmbH, Norderstedt Germany
ISBN: 978-3-656-63398-3

This book at GRIN:

http://www.grin.com/en/e-book/271718/medical-marijuana-and-the-need-for-regulation

Abstract

The issue of medical marijuana has been a challenge to both federal and state authorities for several decades. Recently, with more states legalizing marijuana, this social problem has taken on new proportions mainly because at the Federal level possession even for medical purposes is still an offence. The states that have legalized medical marijuana, have been grappling with problems surrounding mushrooming of dispensaries, an increase in doctor referrals and issues of taxation. Solutions involve streamlining a system for effective registration, distribution and regulation imposition of an effective system of taxation. In addition, medical marijuana needs to be be decriminalized by the federal authorities.

Medical Marijuana and the Need for Regulation

Introduction

The issue of medical marijuana has been with us for decades, however recently this issue has been gaining momentum. According to Cohen (2010), "medical marijuana statute allows practitioners to recommend *Cannabis* for any medical condition, or treatment for such condition, approved by the state health agency...or...[any approved request] submitted by a patient or physician" (p. 659). The proponents for medical marijuana attest that its use by patients who suffer from severe diseases will help to alleviate pain and make their illness more bearable. "In the United States, 16 states and the District of Columbia have legalized marijuana for certain qualifying medical conditions, and efforts are underway to legalize marijuana for medical purposes elsewhere" (Bowles, 2012, p. 9). The states that have legalized are now 18. Furthermore, adults in Colorado and Washington can possess small amounts of marijuana legally. However, regardless of the states' positions, the Federal government has not approved medical marijuana and deems possession of it illegal and has only approved it for research. Furthermore, the Federal Drug Administration has not approved marijuana as being safe and it insists that it has no medical value (Lublum & Ford, 2011). The social issue is that states have failed to design appropriate state regulations to control the distribution and use of medical marijuana. As more states get on board, medical marijuana is becoming more accepted, but there is the potential for abuse of medical referrals, therefore careful assessment, screening and guidelines need to be in place for medical marijuana to serve its intended purpose.

Use of medical marijuana

Marijuana has been used illegally for medical purposes for years, however, in 1996 California legalized medical marijuana, Colorado did similarly in 2000, then other states followed. The marijuana debate shows the conflicting positions of the states and the federal government. One extreme position has supported total legalization, while the Federal law supports prohibition.

Medical Marijuana and the Need for Regulation

Medical marijuana takes a middle ground, restricting its use for medical purposes not clearly defined. The federal law, however, deemed it illegal to possess and to sell marijuana to anyone. "In the debate over medical marijuana, the primary justification advanced by its supporters is that marijuana use, especially by terminally ill patients, mitigates their suffering from unnecessary chronic and unbearable pain that persists until death" (Pfeifer, p. 339). Currently sixteen states have sought a middle position, 'allowing medical marijuana for patients with approved conditions while keeping it illegal for the general population'' (Lublum & Ford, 2011, p. 75).

This conflict left a dilemma where marijuana sellers could be selling it legally in their states but be guilty if found violating federal law. Although still illegal however, President Obama relaxed the enforcement of prosecution for sellers and users of medical marijuana. Medical marijuana has therefore been operating within this grey area of state law and federal law.

As more states take the initiative to legalize medical marijuana the number of loopholes in the system for registration and regulation have been surfacing. According to Reinarman, Numberg, Lanthier & Heddleston, (2011), "Within this grey area between conflicting state and federal laws, the number of patients who have received recommendations for medical marijuana from physicians has continued to grow, albeit by how much remains unknown (p. 129). For example, in 2011, Reinarman et al. found over 1,000 medical marijuana dispensaries operating in California. In Oregon where record keeping for medical marijuana program was required in 2009, there were some 2,983 Oregon licensed physicians who had approved 20, 307 applications for medical marijuana (Reinarman et al, 2011). Reinarman et al. cited that "a medical marijuana advocacy group had estimated that there were well over 200,000 physician-sanctioned medical marijuana patients in California" (p. 120). The system therefore seems to be loosely organized and there is room for improvement in respect to the record keeping procedures.

Furthermore, there is no national registry of patients who are using medical marijuana as the recommended drug for their treatment. In a recent study, Bowles (2012) tried to ascertain the characteristics of persons registered in state-administered medical marijuana programs. Some states did not have a registry while in others registration was voluntary. Because of these constraints (Bowles, 2012) only found "286, 243 people registered for medical marijuana in the United States" (p. 9). In addition, "the majority of persons registered for medical marijuana in

3

the United States appear to be young, male, and registered for severe or chronic pain" (p. 9). The average age of registrants was forty. It seems reasonable to suppose that if medical marijuana is recommended for cancer, glaucoma and other ills that older people would be using it and that the average age of registrants should be much higher. One could argue that there seems to be a half hidden population perhaps because of the cloudy area of uncertainty between the conflicting state and federal legality. Persons might use the 'drug" in secret for recreational use but try to prevent prosecution. However, what is certain is that the number of persons who continue to receive medical marijuana continues to skyrocket although the exact number is not known. To fill this supply and demand dispensaries have continued to mushroom.

The Abuse of Doctor Referrals

The standards by which medical marijuana is to be deemed appropriate are not clearly defined. With the enactment of the medical marijuana law it was expected that the persons who were really ill would get a recommendation from their doctors. However, if only the terminal cancer patients were buying then the hundreds of dispensaries that have sprung up in Colorado for example, would be out of business. According to Ludlum & Ford (2011), as of 2009, there were 80,000 cancer patients in Colorado. What has contributed to the growing increase in medical marijuana patients? Firstly, those who use marijuana as recreational drug would obtain their supply by legal means. Secondly, doctors who provide recommendations do so for financial gain so they are happy to get more patients. Why is there this upsurge in demand for medical marijuana? "The recreational users of marijuana would seek fraudulent means to obtain legal marijuana and avoid the risk of jail" (Ludlum & Ford, 2011, p. 76).

According to Livio (2010), "Denver has 279 medical marijuana dispensaries. By comparison Denver has more dispensaries than Starbucks" (Luvio, 2010). However, many more may be operating without approval. "The web is filled with dispensary ads and an internet search for Denver dispensaries yielded 3, 410, 000 hits on August 31, 2011" (Ludlum & Ford, p. 75). Persons desirous of obtaining medical marijuana need to have a recommendation from a doctor. However, "over 90 percent of patients cite 'severe pain' as a justification" (Livio, 2010). Moreover, the pain does not have to be documented, previously treated, or tied to any diagnosed condition." Persons desired of obtaining medical marijuana are finding means to justify obtaining the drug. According to Segal, 2010, "One physician saw 7000 medical marijuana patients in one year working just three days a week."

4

Criteria for the solution

      Marijuana should be decriminalized but the potential for abuse should be minimized. The solution to this social issue of medical marijuana needs to take into consideration the wishes of the people as represented by the states. The medical value, the dosage, distribution, public safety concerns as reflected by location of dispensaries, economic impact and of course the legality. Scientific studies and/or doctor reports should be available which prove the benefits of medical marijuana. A list of ailments which medical marijuana will cure or alleviate should be available based on scientific studies. Medical marijuana should then be made available like other drugs in pill form or injections or if in plant form the dosage must be streamlined for each specific disease. The relevant dosage that is suggested for particular ailments should be proven scientifically.

Possible Solutions to the Medical Marijuana Issue

      Federal Legalization

      Some have suggested that the way forward might be to propose the outright legalization of marijuana. Recent polls in several states like California, Colorado and Washington show support for marijuana legalization at more than fifty percent. A recent Gallup poll showed for the first time that 50 percent of Americans support legalizing marijuana use (Scott, 2012). However, the government and health professional are opposed to this position. Marijuana lacks FDA approval as a drug. Marijuana is a schedule 1 substance, growing, distribution and possession is a federal crime irrespective of state law. If legalized nationwide easy access by youths and adults for recreational use could lead to psychological problems and persons 'getting high' for recreational reasons. Opponents to federal legalization suggest the lessons we as a nation have learned from the widespread use of cigarettes especially by youths should not be repeated with marijuana. There is potential for abuse by teenagers and recreational users if marijuana is legalized. However, it could be decriminalized.

      Federal Legalization for Medical Use

Currently, according to Federal law marijuana is illegal even for medical use. Many have suggested that it should be legalized for medical purposes only. This seems to be a good solution but in its current form medical marijuana seems to packaged but most often in it plant form. One website (Medical Marijuana) has over one hundred and fifty strains in an alphabetical order with names and the ailments that it is suitable for. Another website pointed to the top sixteen strains. This leads one to ask several questions. Who diagnoses the correct strain for a patient's symptoms? What happens if one strain has a higher content of THC? Moreover, the federal government says that medical marijuana is a front for drug legalization and recreational use. For medical marijuana usage to be effective procedures need to be clearly defined.

State Legalization

Eighteen states and the District of Columbia have legalized marijuana, irrespective of it being illegal according to Federal law. The recreational use of the drug for adults became legal in Colorado and Washington this month. In those states possession of a small amount is legal by state law. However, in relation to medical marijuana the amount permitted under state law varies by state from between 1 ounce to 6 ounces in Delaware, to 8 ounces in California to as high as 24 ounces in Washington. In addition, most states that have legalized marijuana, permit for medical needs, four to seven plants in various stages of maturity. If legalized at the state level for medicinal purposes there seems to be a wide disparity in what different states permit. Could someone leave their state and purchase in another state?

The Best Solution

A Denver medical marijuana dispensary presents a good model of the requirements for distribution. The produce is displayed according to strains and staff members explain the strains and effect. "One staffer, outfitted in blue surgical gloves, describes a strain's chemical properties and genetic history with the same calm, clinical tone of a doctor addressing a patient (Scott, 2012). Each patient visiting the dispensary needs a doctor's referral card. The patient is shown samples while a pharmacist explains the use of the medication. Every procedure in the dispensary is videotaped and monitored by state regulation enforcement agencies.

"We want to make sure there is a legitimate industry to serve this population, so we've created a tight chain of control from seed to sale" (Scott, 2012). In 2010 Colorado lawmakers in an attempt to set up a regulatory system met with representatives of the people and drafted 21 specific rules that state lawmakers passed and Governor Bill Ritter signed into law in 2010.

"In the two years since, nearly 600 medical marijuana centers have been licensed, serving more than 100,000 patients" (Scott, 2012). The system is not perfect but it works. "The Colorado approach is probably the model approach at this point," says Robert Mikos, a law professor at Vanderbilt University who has analyzed medical marijuana laws. "They have much more control of the industry. Other states can look at that, and they can learn from Colorado's experience" (Scott, 2012).

Implementation of the Solution

Step 1: The Department of Health will prepare a list of ailments for which medical marijuana could be prescribed.

Step 2: Identification cards should be issued to qualified patients and primary caregivers. Decide on the penalty for those who obtain cards falsely or prescriptions falsely.

Step 3: Maintain a list of physicians who could issue prescriptions for medical marijuana.

Step 4: Control the purchase amount of marijuana (strains/amount/usage) depending on the patient and the ailment.

Step 5: Maintain a state medical marijuana list of registrants.

Step 6: A pharmacist discuses with patient and orients the patient with the procedure.

Step 7: Create a state board which will decide on penalties for violations, issue fines, control the mandatory registration, commercial cultivation, processing, manufacturing, testing and so on.

Step 8: Establish zoning laws that provide guidelines for the operation of dispensaries. For example: Only one dispensary allowed in an area of 50,000 residents. Dispensaries cannot be located near to schools, parks, playgrounds, main university campus and so on.

Step 9: Provide guidelines for the registering of dispensaries, and for cost of operations, renewal of applications, tax for operations etc.

Step 10: Create a medical marijuana fund for implementation, enforcing and administering all financial aspects of the program.

Step 11: Decide on appropriate tax for business operations. Medical marijuana will undoubtedly provide states with much needed source of revenue.

Conclusion

The people in several states have spoken and others are waiting to make their voices heard. Eighteen states and the District of Columbia have legalized marijuana for medical purposes; however, the Federal government still considers medical marijuana as illegal. An excellent solution to this problem should be to decriminalize medical marijuana but ensure that the states monitor its use stringently. California and Colorado legalized more than a decade ago and their mistakes and how they learned from them have provided guidelines to enable other states to a smoother transition through the process of effective and stricter regulation of medical marijuana.

References

Bowles, D. (2012). Persons registered for medical marijuana in the United States. *Journal of Palliative Medicine.* 15(1) 9-11.

Cohen, P. J. (2010). Medical marijuana 2010: It's time to fix the regulatory vacuum. Journal of law, Medicine & Ethics, 38(3), 654-666.

Livio, S. K. (2010). Tests amid New Jersey's pot law. Gloucester Country Times (New Jersey) (June 6) 1.

Ludlum, M., & Ford, D. (2011). Colorado's 2010 update to the medical marijuana law: Three problems, three solutions. 2011 Mustang Journal of Law and Legal Studies, 73-80.

Medical Marijuana. http://medicalmarijuana.com/medical-marijuana-strains-1

Pfeifer, D. J. (2011). Smoking gun: The moral and legal struggle for medical marijuana. Touro Law Review, 27, 339-377.

Reinarman, C., Numberg, M., Lanthier, F., & Heddleston, M. (2011). Who are medical marijuana patients? Population characteristics from nine California assessment clinics. *Journal of Psychoactive Drugs*, 43(2), 128-135.

Scott, D. (2012). Medical marijuana: have states finally learned how to regulate it? Governing. (Aug. 01)

Segal, D. (2010). When capitalism meets cannabis. *New York Times*. (June 27) 3.